THE POWER TO HEAL MYSELF

by

Betty Jean Wall

ISBN 978-0-578-02743-2

Acknowledgments

Everyone is my teacher. Thank you. You have been kind, generous, and honest. You allowed me to cry. You have accepted me as I am. You have loved me. You have taught me in classes. You, I have had the privilege of touching. You have touched me. You spend time with me. You have encouraged me to write this book. You have read over the book in various stages of its development. You are all the **Self, eternal Beings.** I love each of you, my- self. With you, my life is rich, abundant with love, laughter and fun. Thank you, thank you, thank you.

Also by or edited by Betty Jean Wall

Transport of Ions and Water in Animals, 1977
    B.L. Gupta, R.B. Moreton, J.L. Oschman and B.J.Wall, eds.

Going Through God, 1982, 2006

Clandestine Acclamations, 2006, by Reta Simpson, ed. by Betty Jean Wall

Riplion, Dancing through the spiral, 2007, by Barbara Gates Burwell and Betty Jean Wall

Table of Contents

Preface

The suggestions for helping oneself in the following pages are inspired from the self help books that Mary Burmeister published in 1981 and 1985 (see Burmeister, Mary, 1985a, 1981, 1985b, *Introducing Jin Shin Jyutsu Is, Book I, II, III*. I am also inspired from participating in classes taught by Mary Burmeister and other instructors of Jin Shin Jyutsu, Rolfing, Rolfing Movement, Tuina, Chi Kung, Healing Touch, and Trauma Energetics. I have been using the exercises daily since 1981. My studies in correlating structure and function, observing human behavior (including my own), contributed to understanding how the body works and how the whole person behaves in the world. We are each in a lifelong class in the art of living.

Mary Burmeister was an American born of Japanese parents. While she was a young adult in Japan teaching English, she met Jiro Murai, a Master and teacher who had discovered an ancient healing art. Over time this art became known as "Jin Shin Jyutsu, the Art of Knowing or Helping Myself." Master Murai asked Mary if she wanted to bring a gift back to the United States, and she said "Yes." That gift is the art of Jin Shin Jyutsu. She studied with Master Murai for a number of years before she came back home to the United States. She continued her studies for years before she started sharing her understanding with others. Mary taught classes and gave treatments to many people over the years. Her spirit lives on although her body has returned to the earth. She continues to inspire me and many others daily as we practice the loving art of Jin Shin Jyutsu.

I have also been inspired by Haruki Kato of Japan who was a student of Master Jiro Murai after Mary returned to the United States. Kato Sensai has also taught classes for Jin Shin Jyutsu students.

Jin Shin Jyutsu classes are being taught and are open to anyone who wants to learn. Contact www.jsjinc.net for more information about classes or for Mary Burmeister's self help books.

Rolfing is about structural integration of the body. It was developed by Ida P. Rolf, a biochemist, who wanted to find help for her son. She recognized the importance of freeing the body of its structural constrictions, so that we could move and function better, be supported by the earth and gravity. When the body is structurally aligned, we also function better emotionally and mentally. We are then in touch with our spirit, our soul. We can then fulfill our life's purpose. When we have integrity in life, we tell the truth, we act in a conscious way and we are awake. The body knows the truth, and will respond to untruth by shortening its muscles even if the mind ignores the lie. The Rolf Institute of Structural Integration teaches classes and can be reached at www.rolf.org for information. The Guild for Structural Integration also teaches classes and can be reached at www.rolfguild.org.

I am always thankful that the course of my life has been changed by these two pioneers, Mary Burmeister and Ida Rolf. I feel I am fulfilling my life's purpose by getting to know myself and wake up. Working with people gives me joy, keeps me learning and understanding that life is about being.

My life did not always feel so alive. I was so ignorant of myself for many years, and now I know myself more every day. I offer and share these suggestions in this book to you as a friend who has happily prepared a dish for you to enjoy. You know more about yourself than anyone else does. I do not have all the answers.

Many of you could write such a book as I have, each with your own wisdom and sense of fun. Perhaps this will encourage you to share what you want to share. This book is about what you can do to facilitate healing. There are many more elements that comprise an overall healthy life, such as spending time with loved ones, finding one's life work, being in nature, growing/preparing one's food, exercising, quieting the mind, realizing the SELF, living and dying consciously.

Putting this book together has been a joyful project, fun at every step. You may contact me at www.bettyjeanwall.com

Betty Jean Wall

Woods Hole, MA
February 18, 2009

INTRODUCTION

Each of us has the power to heal within ourselves. Our attitudes, our thoughts can be changed to those of harmony. The physical body is the manifestation of past actions, attitudes, and thoughts. Within this life I can heal myself. You can heal yourself. We have the power. We let go of the past and be in the present. Exhale all that we no longer need. Affirm health in what we think and speak.

BASIC PRINCIPLES OF LIFE

We are love.

We are CONSCIOUSNESS.

We are already enlightened.

We just have to show up and be present.

We are here to serve and to share.

We are joy, laughter, happiness and FUN.

In addition to nurturing each other with food, we can nurture each other's souls by being kind, compassionate, forgiving. We are all reflections of each other.

SILENCE

Spending time in silence has helped me to be more careful with the words I speak and the thoughts I think. Being silent allows me time to face myself, to reflect, to change my attitude, to show me what I need to change in my own behavior. If I am judging or criticizing someone's behavior, it is the mind's FEAR which is judging and criticizing. Stop the mind's constant chatter. By quieting the mind, then we can be open to learning, then we can really hear. The most profound teachings are beyond words and are taught and learned in silence. Gandhi had a weekly 24 hour silence.

Spending time together in Silence is sacred.

LISTENING

We each want to be heard.

"HOW DO I LISTEN?

How
Do I
Listen to Others?
As if everyone were my Master
Speaking to me
His
Cherished
Last
Words."

From the Penguin publication *The Gift, Poems by Hafiz*, copyright 1999 Daniel Ladinsky and used with his permission.

PRACTICING

Life is practice. Practice listening. Practice kindness. In order to be peace, we have to practice peace. We have to practice choosing peace instead of choosing to be right. In each situation, we have to practice non-violence in thoughts, words, and actions, live from soul.

We must forgive. Even as our hearts are breaking, we are to perceive everyone as a kind loving person. We can bring forth kindness in each other.

We are all souls having a life on earth. We are human beings all joined together, all interconnected. We each feel the pain of suffering of each other.

Quiet the mind, forgive, and be compassionate.
Be **peace**.

EXERCISES

Upon awakening to a new day, allow the feeling of joy to flow over your whole being and smile. Give thanks for another day. Then start using the exercises listed below.

Mudras

Mudras are special positions of the hands or body which are used to bring about harmony and healing. Mudras have been used for thousands of years all over the world. You may read more about the history of mudras from the book *Mudras, Yoga in your hands*, by Gertrud Hirschi, 2000.

The following pages (pp.9-23, Figs. 1-10) show hand positions which help to heal, from Burmeister, Mary, 1985b, *Introducing Jin Shin Jyutsu Is*, Book III, pp.9-17, and Hirschi, 2000.

While holding each hand position slowly let go of several deep breaths.

By counting each breath, the mind is focused on counting and is thus prevented from worrying or obsessing. So at least during the time of counting, the mind is not getting into trouble. It is a way of quieting the mind.

Each hand position can be used anytime and for as long as you want.

Hand Positions

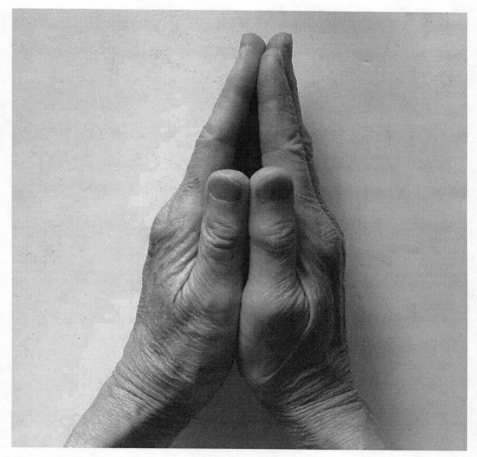

Figure 1) Place the palms together in front of the heart.

This hand position creates harmony, silence, peace, calmness. This mudra harmonizes left and right brain. It is used in many countries when greeting people. It is used to show reverence and gratitude.

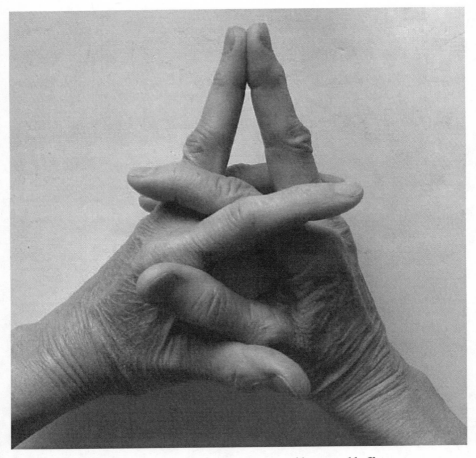

Figure 2) Place palms together, allow all fingers to intertwine except for middle fingers which remain straight.

This position brings about calmness and harmony. It releases daily tension from head, lungs, digestive functions, abdomen and legs. It aids exhaling and letting go.

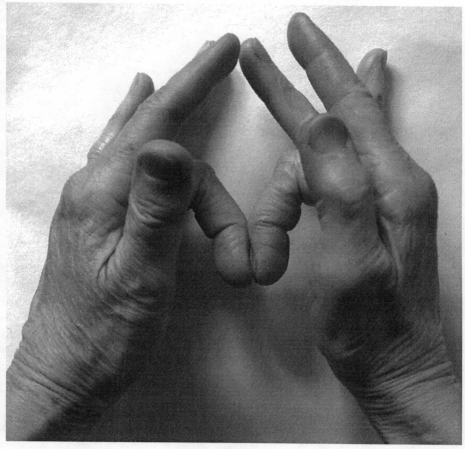

Figure 3) Place middle fingernails together while keeping other fingers extended.

This position relieves back tension and helps inhale of breath especially with asthmatic conditions.

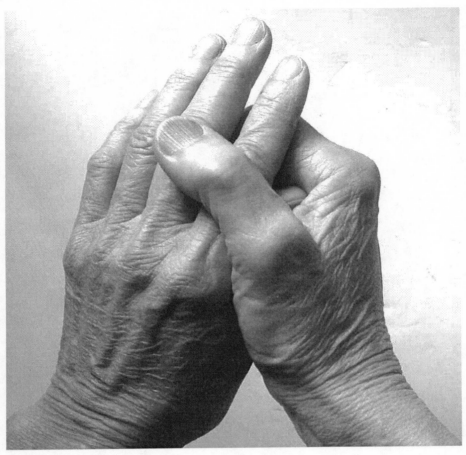

Figure 4 a) With left hand palm down, place right hand around left middle finger, left index finger and left thumb with right thumb on back side of left fingers.

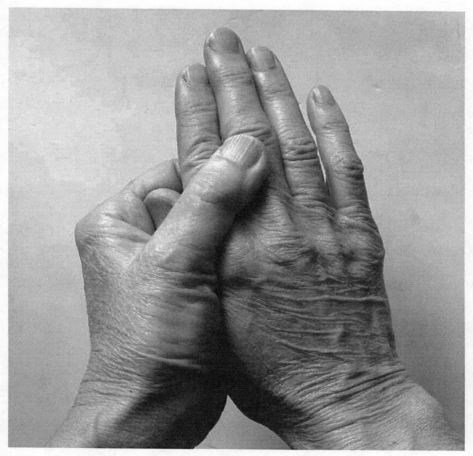

Figure 4 b) With right hand palm down, place left hand around right middle finger, left index finger and left thumb with left thumb on back side of right hand.

This hand position shown in Figures 4 a, b, releases tension in back, helps breathing, lets go of fatigue, releases worry, fear and anger.

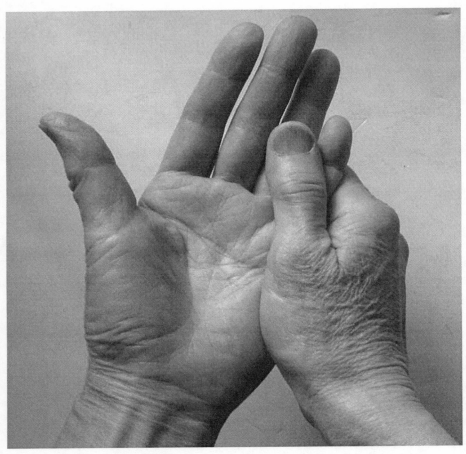

Figure 5 a) With left hand palm up, place right hand around left little finger and left ring finger.

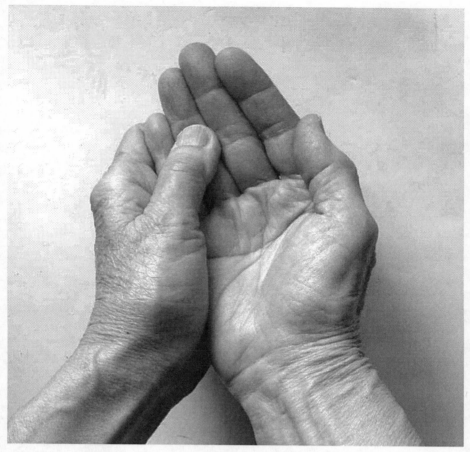

Figure 5 b) With right hand palm up, place left hand around right little finger and right ring finger.

This hand position shown in Figures 5 a, b, energizes body, energizes bladder, small intestine, heart and spleen, calms nerves, helps vascular system, releases sadness and helps breathing. It aids sleep and lessens depression.

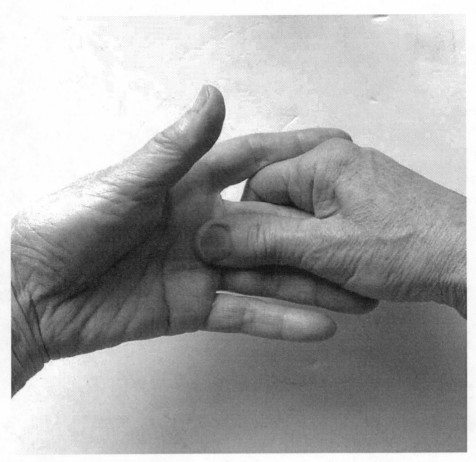

Figure 6 a) With left hand palm up, place right hand around left middle finger with right thumb on palm side of left middle finger.

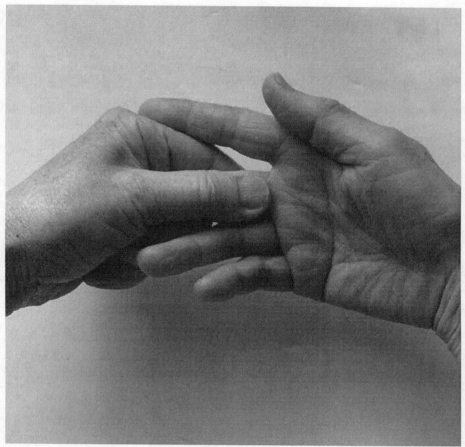

Figure 6 b) With right hand palm up, place left hand around right middle finger with left thumb on palm side of right middle finger.

This hand position shown in Figures 6 a, b, helps to release tension from whole body and helps exhale of breath, eyes, fatigue and frustration.

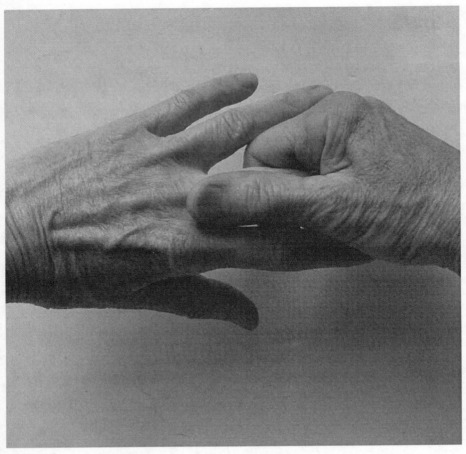

Figure 7 a) With left hand palm down, place right hand around left middle finger with right thumb on back side of left middle finger.

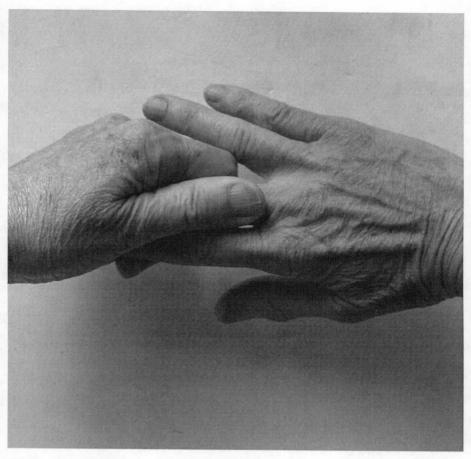

Figure 7 b) With right hand palm down, place left hand around right middle finger with left thumb on back side of right middle finger.

This hand position shown in Figures 7 a, b, helps to energize whole body, helps inhale of breath, hearing, feet and alertness.

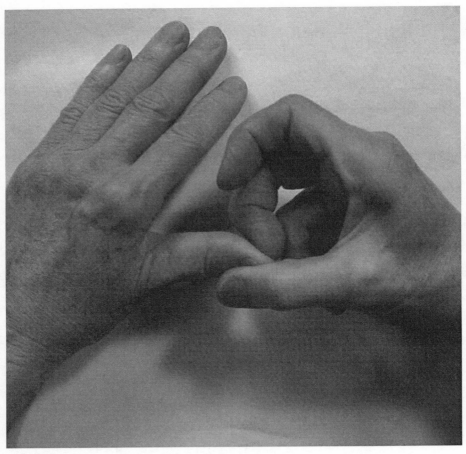

Figure 8 a) Place right thumb over right middle fingernail. Slip left thumb between right thumb and right middle finger.

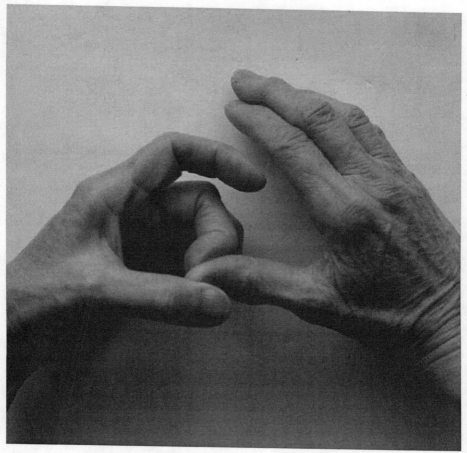

Figure 8 b) Place left thumb over left middle fingernail. Slip right thumb between left thumb and left middle finger.

This hand position shown in Figures 8 a, b, helps to energize functions of body, to let go of fatigue, to let go of craving for sugar, helps with complexion and jet lag. Use when feeling uneasy or temperamental.

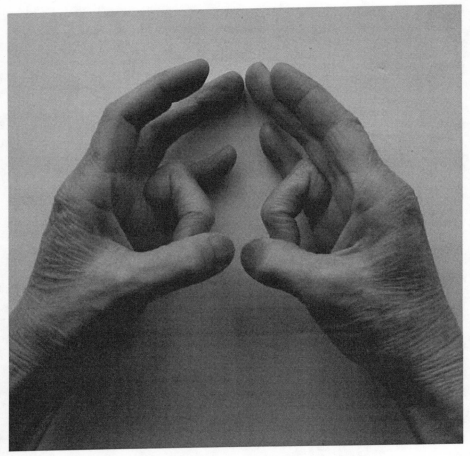

Figure 9) Place thumb over ring fingernail.

This hand position helps breathing when short of breath while exercising or going to high altitudes. It helps ear, skin and balances emotions. Use when feeling clumsy.

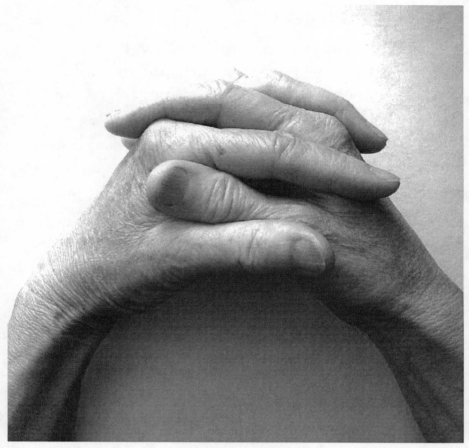

Figure 10) Intertwine fingers with palms facing each other, allow right thumb to rest between left thumb and left index finger.

This hand position helps with mental alertness, helps to wake up in the morning and helps hormonal balance.

Changing Attitudes

The following finger sequences are from Burmeister, Mary, 1985a, *Introducing Jin Shin Jyutsu Is*, Book I, pp.21-36, "Getting to KNOW (Help) MYSELF- ATTITUDES."

These sequences help us to change the attitudes of: Worry, Fear, Anger, Sadness, and Pretense. We can change these attitudes that keep us from being present and happy. Happiness is our natural state. Yet too much sadness will cover up the happiness which is within us. Too much worry and fear will keep us from being present and wear down the body of its strength. Too much anger will make us explode and lose the source of our power. Too much pretense or "trying to be perfect" will keep us from being who we really are. By holding the fingers we can start changing these attitudes. By holding the fingers everyday, we can transform our attitudes as well as our lives. By changing ourselves, we allow those around us to change. Harmony and peace within will spread to others around us.

We are each energy and matter. The energy flows throughout the body as invisible lines of energy spiraling up and down the physical body, going through every organ and tissue, every finger and toe, in organized pathways. By holding the fingers or holding the body in different places we facilitate the energy moving in harmony through these pathways.

Attitude: Worry

Worrying also includes a variety of behavior.

We may constantly think about an upcoming event and even though we have all the preparations in order, we keep changing our minds about some of the details.

We may constantly tell our children to make good grades in school.

We may schedule our time so that we are rushed to be on time for our activities, or we may show up hours early for an event.

We feel depressed, or irritable, out of sorts, insecure or nervous.

We use the word "hate" for expressing ourselves about a lot of things in our lives.

We wake up at night and cannot stop thinking about an upcoming talk, test, interview or the next day, etc.

We have a stomach ache, or have trouble breathing, pant, or have tensed up shoulders, neck and back.

We are eating constantly even though we are not hungry. We crave sweets. We feel bloated.

We may constantly lick the lips, move the tongue around the mouth, swallow, twirl the hair, scratch the skin, or otherwise be moving some part of the body.

We often anticipate "something going wrong" with any plan and are busy thinking of alternatives "just in case."

Let Go of WORRY

The following sequence in Figures 11 a, b, c, for right hand and Figures 12 a, b, c, for left hand helps to let go of worry, anxiety, and obsession. This sequence also helps stomach and spleen functions.

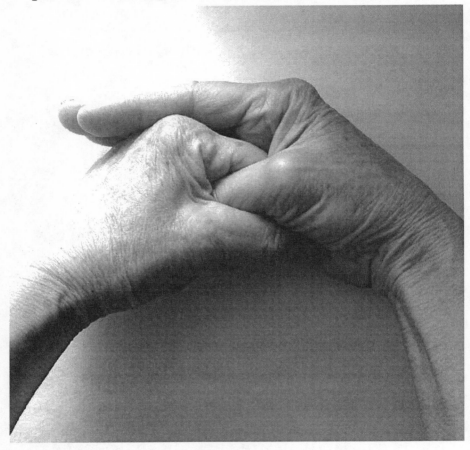

Figure 11 a) Place left hand around right thumb while slowly letting go of several deep breaths.

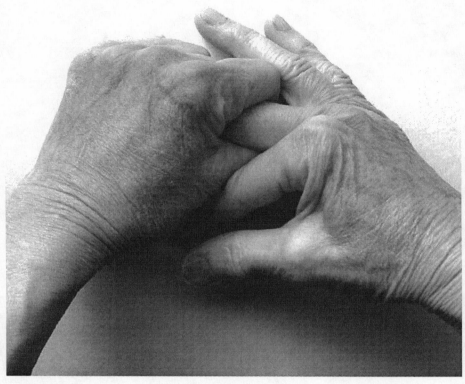

Figure 11 b) Place left hand around right middle finger while slowly letting go of several deep breaths.

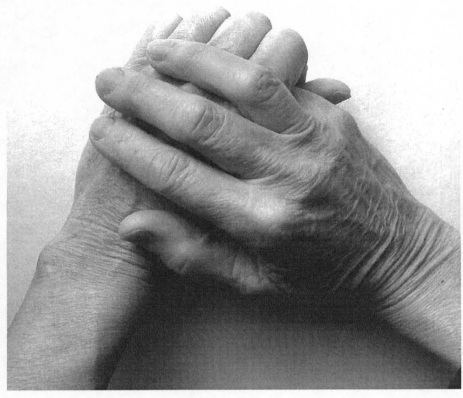

Figure 11c) Place left hand around right little finger while slowly letting go of several deep breaths.

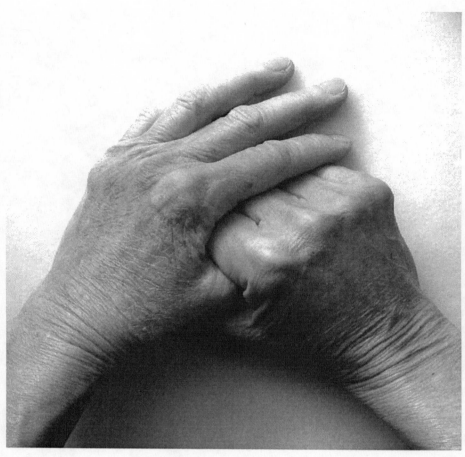

Figure 12 a) Place right hand around left thumb while slowly letting go of several deep breaths.

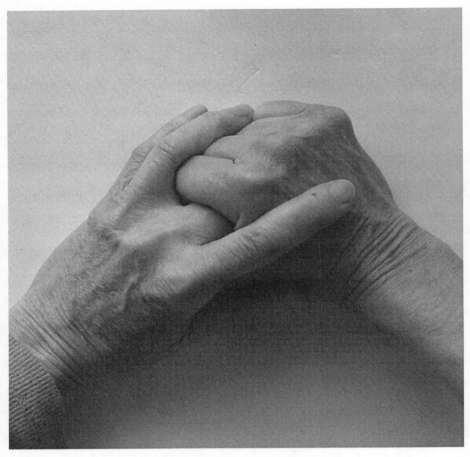

Figure 12 b) Place right hand around left middle finger while slowly letting go of several deep breaths.

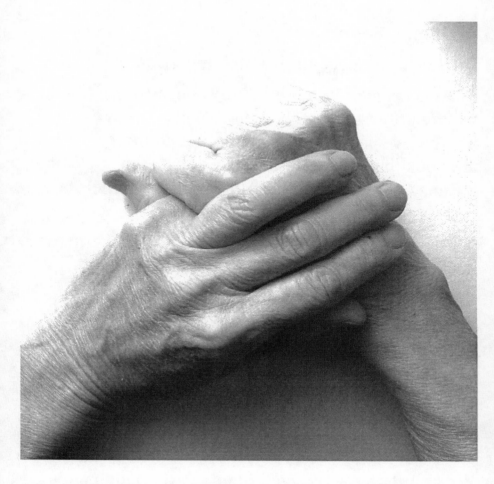

Figure 12 c) Place right hand around left little finger while slowly letting go of several deep breaths.

The attitude of worry can use up much of our time and energy. When we worry we are imagining something we do not want, however, if we imagine or picture something long enough, we are bringing it into existence. So we would be better off to imagine what we want.

Attitude: Fear

Below are behaviors which represent fear.

We are constantly buying things because we think we are going to run out even though we have plenty of what we are buying. We hold onto things. We are constipated. We accumulate vast sums of money because we are afraid we might end up homeless in our old age.

When company is coming we cook too much food because we are afraid we will not have enough.

We crave salt.

We try to manage the lives of others: our spouses, partners, or friends by telling them how to or when to do something, what to do, how to be or what to wear. We are super critical of our own and of other people's appearance.

We are afraid to cry, thinking we would fall apart.

We belittle ourselves and others in our language.

We cannot accept a compliment.

We want revenge.

We feel unloved.

We say "Yes" when we really want to say "No." We do not speak with clarity, nor do we tell the truth.

We do not keep our commitments.

We cannot talk of death or face our own death.

Let go of FEAR

The following sequence in Figures 13 a, b, c, for right hand and Figures 14 a, b, c, for left hand helps to eliminate FEAR. This sequence also helps bladder and kidney functions.

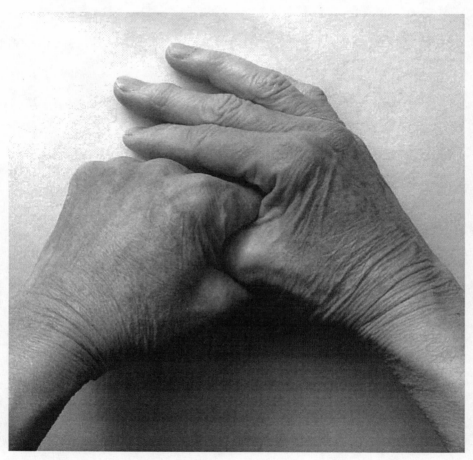

Figure 13 a) Place left hand around right thumb while slowly letting go of several deep breaths.

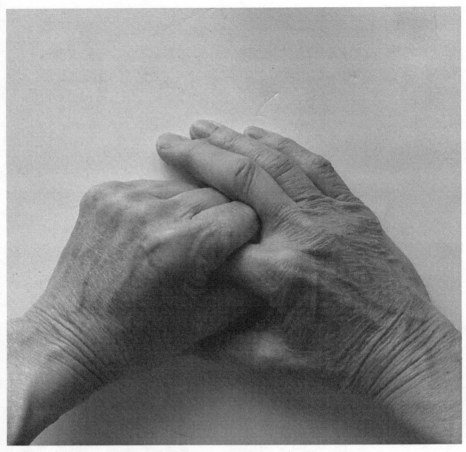

Figure 13 b) Place left hand around right index finger while slowly letting go of several deep breaths.

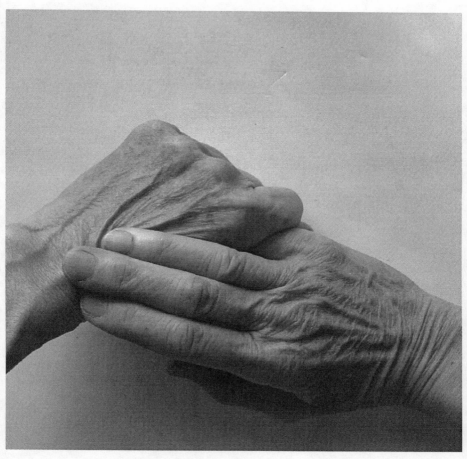

Figure 13 c) Place left hand around right little finger while slowly letting go of several deep breaths.

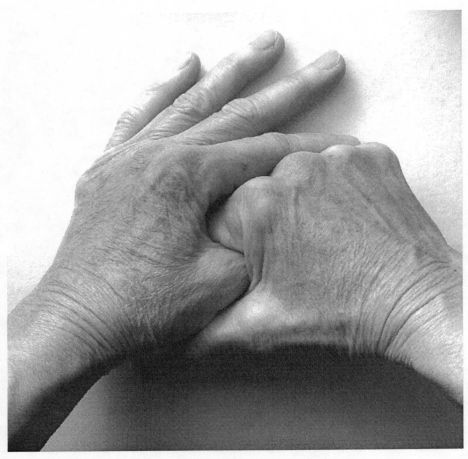

Figure 14 a) Place right hand around left thumb while slowly letting go of several deep breaths.

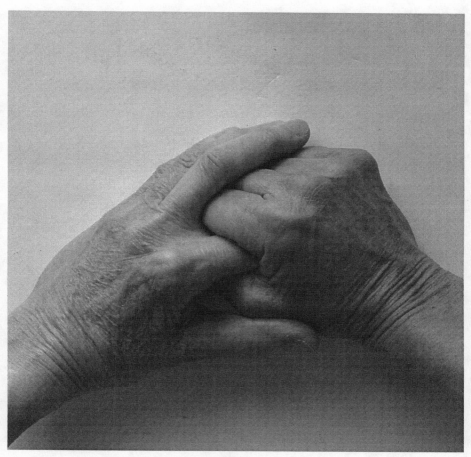

Figure 14 b) Place right hand around left index finger while slowly letting go of several deep breaths.

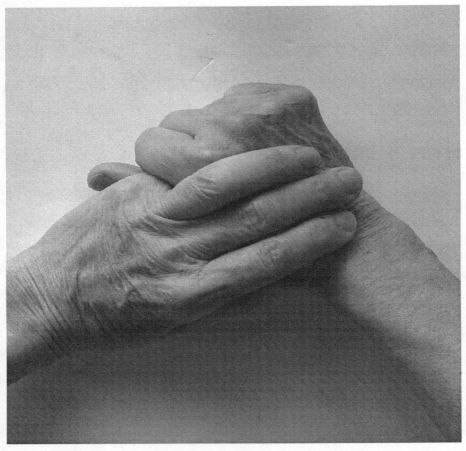

Figure 14 c) Place right hand around left little finger while slowly letting go of several deep breaths.

Dr. Alexis Carrel, *Man, the Unknown,* says that "Where the disease itself takes the lives of hundreds, it is perhaps true that fear claims victims by the thousands. Thought becomes obviously the most important factor of cure and control under such situations….Fear is paralyzing in its effects." From Heline, Corrine, 1940, *Occult Anatomy and the Bible,* p.16. Fear stresses all functions of body. Exhale and let go of fear.

Attitude: Anger

The following behaviors are examples of anger.

We clench our jaws or our fists and say to ourselves or to the other driver something negative about their driving.

We are resentful of our husband/wife/friend being too busy to spend time with the children/me.

We wish that someone would show appreciation for or acknowledge what we do for them.

We speak with a high pitched and strained voice.

We feel frustrated.

We are complaining all the time.

We do not speak up.

Letting go of ANGER

The following sequence in Figures 15 a, b, c, for right hand and Figures 16 a, b, c, for left hand helps to eliminate ANGER. This sequence also helps liver and gall bladder functions.

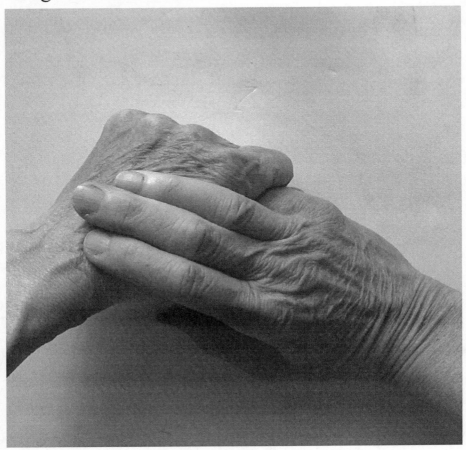

Figure 15 a) Place left hand around right little finger while slowly letting go of several deep breaths.

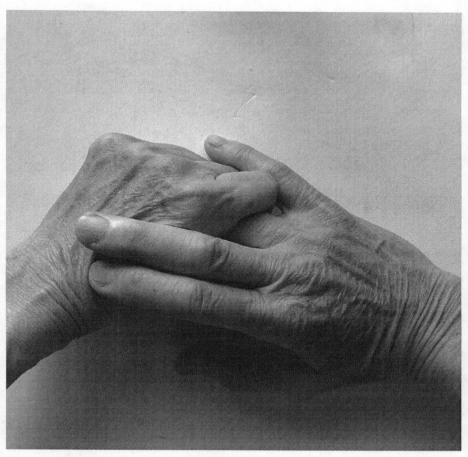

Figure 15 b) Place left hand around right ring finger while slowly letting go of several deep breaths.

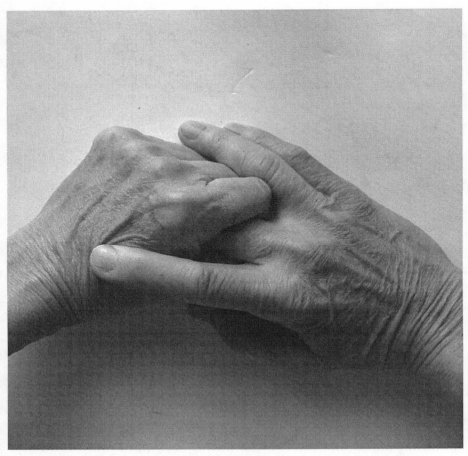

Figure 15 c) Place left hand around right middle finger while slowly letting go of several deep breaths.

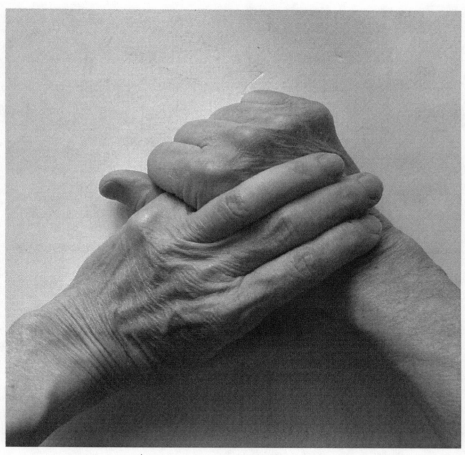

Figure 16 a) Place right hand around left little finger while slowly letting go of several deep breaths.

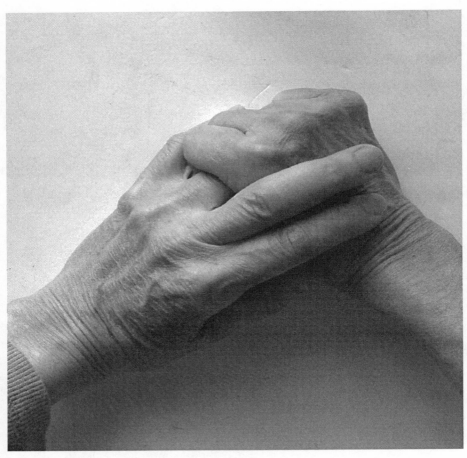

Figure 16 b) Place right hand around left ring finger while slowly letting go of several deep breaths.

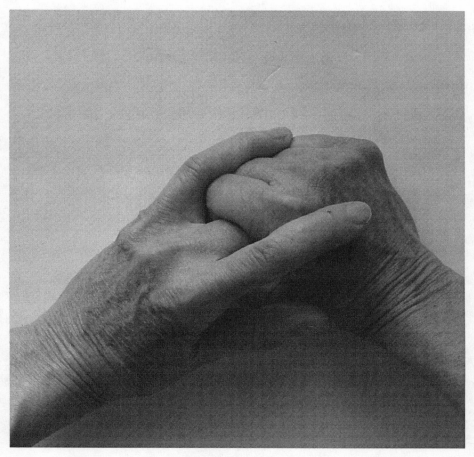

Figure 16 c) Place right hand around left middle finger while slowly letting go of several deep breaths.

Pent up anger interferes with our ability to think and see clearly and, like fear, anger stresses our immune system. Holding this sequence helps us to let go of tensions which cause anger.

Attitude: Sadness

The following behaviors are examples of sadness.

The voice is weepy.

We keep thinking of someone who has died/moved away years ago and wish they were still here.

We have had too many changes in one year: death of a loved one, we have moved or changed/lost the job.

We have had one cold after another.

We have developed trouble with the colon.

We are crying at a moment's notice; almost anything will make us cry.

We just want to be lazy. We feel like a sorry mess and do not want to go out of our room/house. We are immobilized.

We are uncomfortable around someone who is crying.

Letting go of SADNESS

The following sequence in Figures 17 a, b, c, d, for right hand and Figures 18 a, b, c, d, for left hand helps let go of sadness. The sequence also helps lung and large intestine functions.

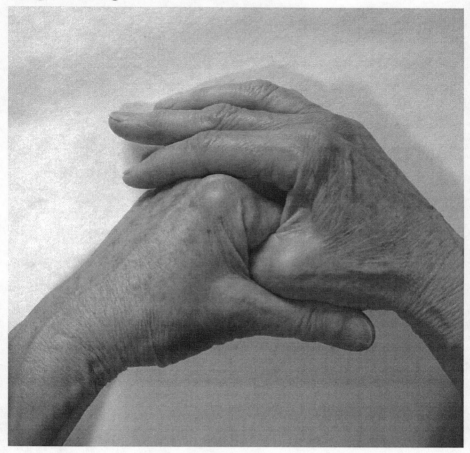

Figure 17 a) Place left hand around right thumb while slowly letting go of several deep breaths.

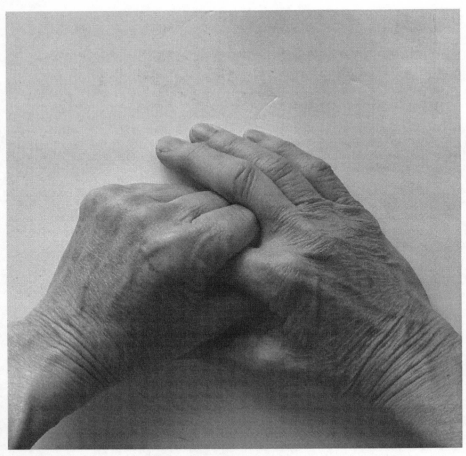

Figure 17 b) Place left hand around right index finger while slowly letting go of several deep breaths.

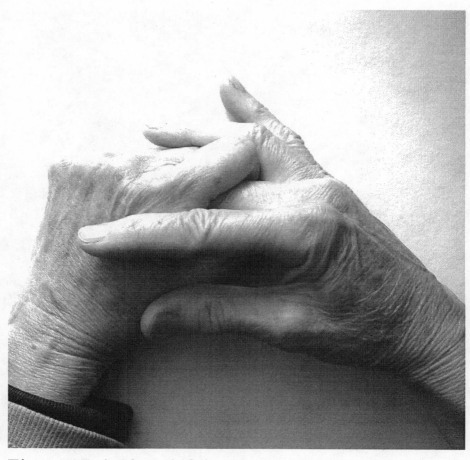

Figure 17 c) Place left hand around right middle finger while slowly letting go of several deep breaths.

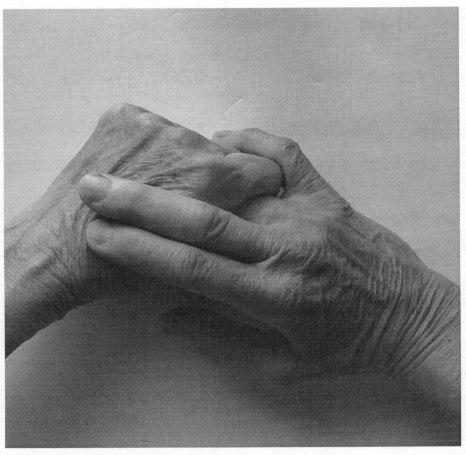

Figure 17 d) Place left hand around right ring finger while slowly letting go of several deep breaths.

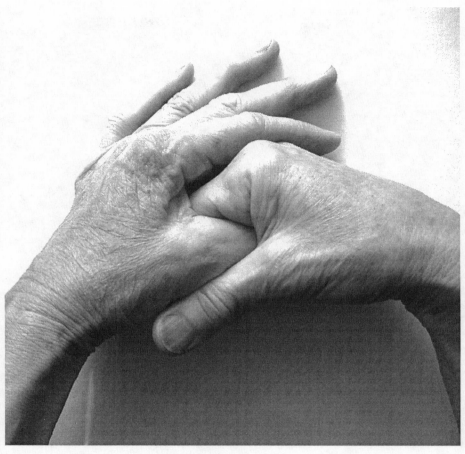

Figure 18 a) Place right hand around left thumb while slowly letting go of several deep breaths.

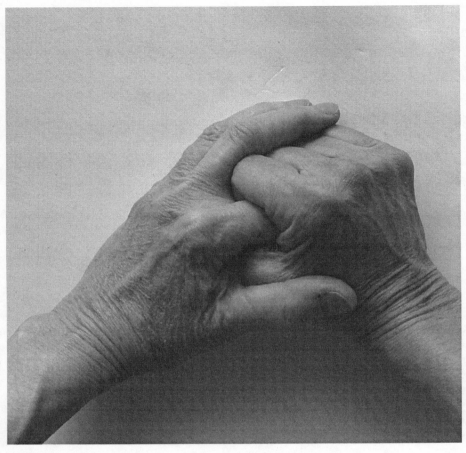

Figure 18 b) Place right hand around left index finger while slowly letting go of several deep breaths.

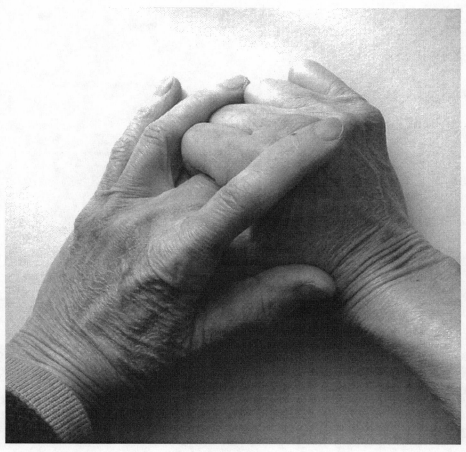

Figure 18 c) Place right hand around left middle finger while slowly letting go of several deep breaths.

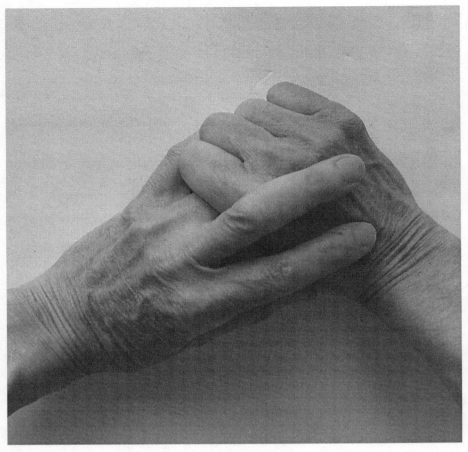

Figure 18 d) Place right hand around left ring finger while slowly letting go of several deep breaths.

Long time sadness dampens our happiness to the point that every single cell is crying and losing its ability to maintain its identity, cutting off communication with its neighboring cells. As the wave of sadness comes, exhale to let it wash out of the body, and let every cell smile.

Attitude: Pretense

The following behaviors are examples of pretense.

We go to the funeral of our dear loved one and we talk/smile as if nothing has happened when on the inside we are crying.

We really feel like screaming but we clench our jaws and hold it in.

We think we are fooling the others by our cheerfulness when we really feel disappointed because we did not pass the exam or get the job or win the race.

We are always trying to be perfect.

We dress to appear much older or younger than what we really are.

We think we need to be different from the way we are.

We do not speak to certain people because we feel we are better or more important than they are.

We find ourselves using the word "try" in our sentences.

Letting go of PRETENSE

The following sequence in Figures 19 a, b, for right hand and Figures 20 a, b, for left hand helps to let go of pretense or "trying to," laughing on the outside, crying on the inside. This sequence also helps heart and small intestine functions.

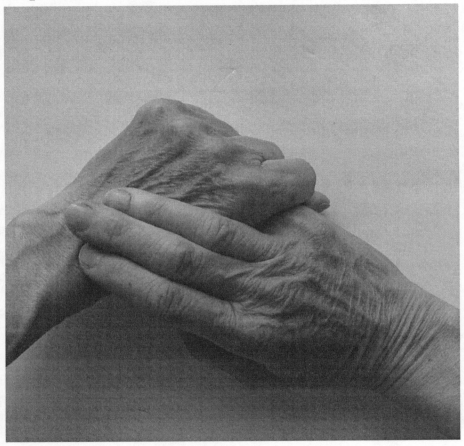

Figure 19 a) Place left hand around right little finger while slowly letting go of several deep breaths.

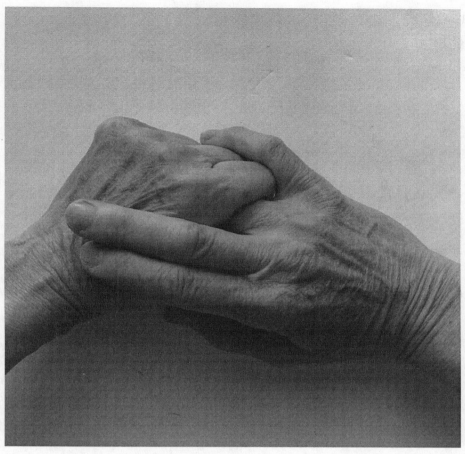

Figure 19 b) Place left hand around right ring finger while slowly letting go of several deep breaths.

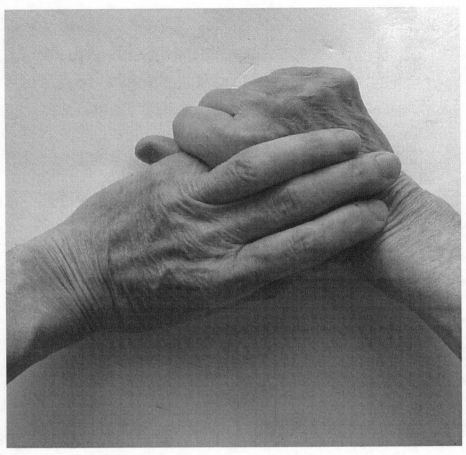

Figure 20 a) Place right hand around left little finger while slowly letting go of several deep breaths.

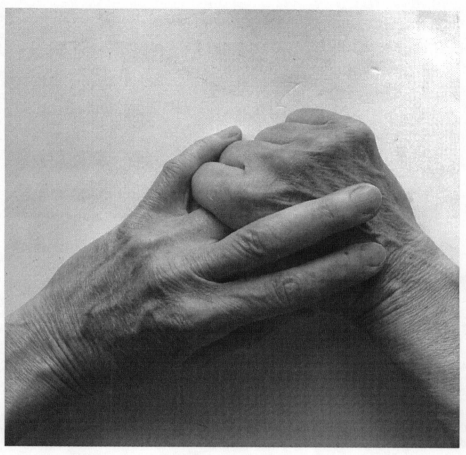

Figure 20 b) Place right hand around left ring finger while slowly letting go of several deep breaths.

I have pretended. I have laughed on the outside while I cried on the inside. We pretend when we are afraid that who we are and the way we are is not all right. We judge ourselves to be lacking in some way. A life of pretense is a life missed, of not being present. Let go of FEAR. Each of us is unique. Let us be who we truly are, magnificent creatures. Let us live from our soul, as loving compassionate human beings.

If you do not have time to go through the sequences of holding the fingers, you can just hold the thumb for worry, the index finger for fear, the middle finger for anger, the ring finger for sadness, and the little finger for pretense. Hold each finger for 3 minutes to help harmonize all the functions of the body.

Your life may be so busy that you do not have 30 minutes in a day to hold the fingers, then just hold the center of the palm to help everything or hold any finger of your choice. If that is not possible, just be present for each breath. When we can no longer hold the fingers, there is still the breath.

Main Central

The beginning of this life starts in the womb when the sperm and egg combine. Invisible energy starts flowing in the embryo to orient the cells during cell division in forming the body, with head at one end and feet at the other end. This is the basis of our form, first we are energy, and then we are matter.

The first energy to flow through the body is up the midline of the back and down the midline of the front. This basic energetic flow is continuous throughout our whole lives as long as we are living. When it stops, the body dies. This basic energy is called the "Main Central." The next 2 pages show how we can keep the Main Central clear.

Harmonizing whole body with Main Central from Burmeister, 1985a, pp.15-17, see Figure 21 next page:

Step 1: While lying down, place right hand on top of head (stays here until last step).

Place left hand between eyebrows. Revitalizes body, helps memory, helps sleep.

Step 2: Place left hand on tip of nose. Helps reproductive system, stomach, balances appetite.

Step 3: Place left hand in notch between collar bones. Balances reproductive and creative functions, helps thyroid and parathyroid.

Step 4: Place left hand on center of sternum (breast bone). Helps youthfulness, immune system, thymus, breathing, hips.

Step 5: Place left hand at tip of sternum (solar plexus area). Helps digestion, vision, and joints, revitalizes body energy.

Step 6: Place left hand 1 inch above navel. Helps breathing and reproductive function.

Step 7: Place left hand on pubic bone. Helps spine, helps letting go of tensions in head, chest and abdomen.

Last step: Place right hand on tail bone. Helps circulation of legs and feet, energizes back.

While in each position slowly breathe out and in for several deep breaths.

Main Central

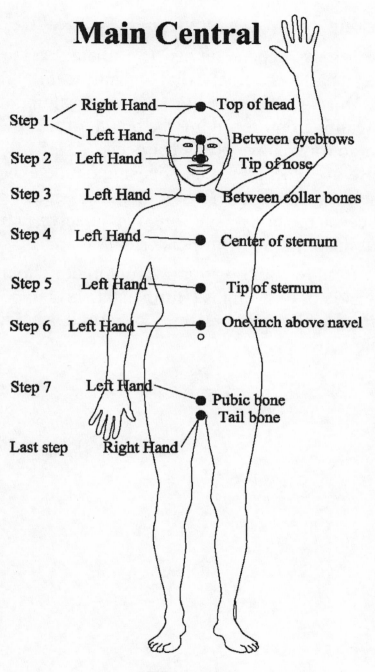

Right Hand — Top of head

Step 1

Left Hand — Between eyebrows

Step 2   Left Hand — Tip of nose

Step 3   Left Hand — Between collar bones

Step 4   Left Hand — Center of sternum

Step 5   Left Hand — Tip of sternum

Step 6   Left Hand — One inch above navel

Step 7   Left Hand

Pubic bone
Tail bone

Last step   Right Hand

Figure 21

Breathing

In birth, we depend on the first inhale. At the end of life on earth, the final exhale means death of the body. During our whole lives we are breathing in and breathing out, receiving the breath of life and letting go of what we no longer need. A daily exercise of 36 deep breaths, focusing on the exhale, will help us to be conscious of the gift of each breath and cleanse the body. We can give ourselves a big hug while breathing (Burmeister, 1985b, p.41).

For trouble with breathing, coughing or choking, hold inside of mid-thighs (Burmeister, 1985a, p. 51) with both hands until breathing is normal, see Figure 22 below.

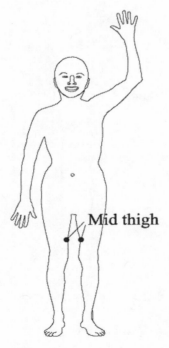

Mid thigh

Figure 22

Release Shoulders

Right side: Place the left hand over the right shoulder; place the right hand on the right sit bone (ischial tuberosity) from Burmeister, 1985a, p52, see Figure 23 below.

Left side: Place right hand over left shoulder; place left hand on the left sit bone.

This combination releases tension, "excess baggage," in each shoulder. It also helps relieve abdominal tension, cramps, or pain, and helps exhale of breath.

Exhale, clear the mind, then we can "**Be still and know**," if we are still, we will know the **Self**.

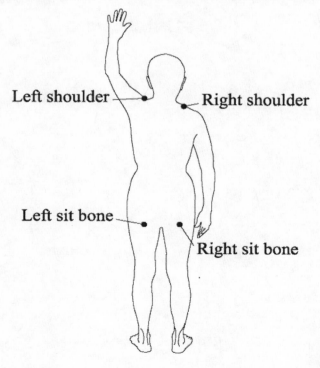

Left shoulder

Right shoulder

Left sit bone

Right sit bone

Figure 23

Release shoulders and back

Right side: Place left hand over right shoulder; place right hand on right groin area (where leg joins body), Burmeister, 1981, see Figure 24 below.

Left side: Place right hand over left shoulder; place left hand on left groin area.

This position helps to release tension in each shoulder. It also helps relieve back tension and helps inhale of breath.

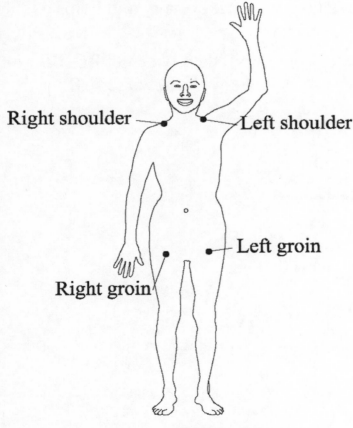

Figure 24

By holding left shoulder and left sit bone, and then left shoulder and left groin, we harmonize the left side front and back. By holding the right shoulder and right sit bone, and then right shoulder and right groin, we harmonize the right side front and back.

Rejuvenate

Placing right hand on right sit bone and left hand on left sit bone (Burmeister, 1985a, 1981) will help to rejuvenate, see Figure 23. This position is helpful to calm the body after you have had some physical exercise. However, on those days when you cannot exercise physically, just place the hands on the sit bones for 20 minutes to quietly rejuvenate. This position has also helped with people who want to lose weight, place the hands on the sit bones for 20 minutes a day, and the pounds will melt away.

Legs

Place right hand on right groin area (Burmeister, 1981) to help right leg, knee, and foot, see Figure 24.

Place left hand on left groin area to help left leg, knee, and foot.

Placing the hands on the groin area also helps to uncover the laughter and joy within us.

For neck tension, also for **back tension**, from Burmeister, 1985a, p.48. <u>Right neck and back</u>: With left hand under neck, hold the right side of neck. With right hand hold coccyx (tail bone), then back of right knee, then outside of right ankle, and then right little toe. See Figure 25 below:

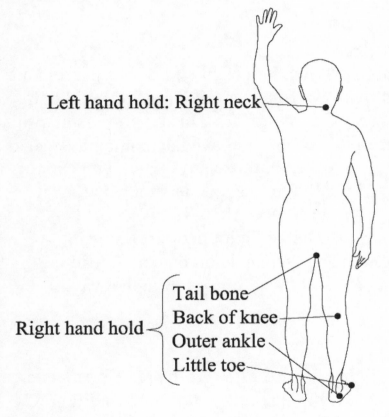

Left hand hold: Right neck

Right hand hold ⎰ Tail bone
⎱ Back of knee
Outer ankle
Little toe

Figure 25

This sequence can be done sitting up although lying down may allow neck and back muscles to relax more easily.

<u>Left neck and back</u>: With right hand under neck, hold the left side of neck. With left hand hold tail bone, then back of left knee, then outside of left ankle, then left little toe.

This sequence shown in Figure 25 also helps with discomfort in head, migraine headaches, epilepsy, balance mental state, bloody nose, eyes, hip, incontinence, back, knee, muscle spasms in calf, weakness in legs, itching, and fear.

For stomach ache

Hold insides of mid-thighs, see Figure 22. See also Figure 26 below, from Burmeister, 1985a, pp.43-44.

The sequence shown in Figure 26 can be used to harmonize any stomach imbalances, to balance appetite, to clear the head, the nose, for dry mouth or lips, complexion, skin tags, neck and throat issues, abdominal bloat or cramping, addictions, back, knee, breast, groin, ankle or foot discomforts.

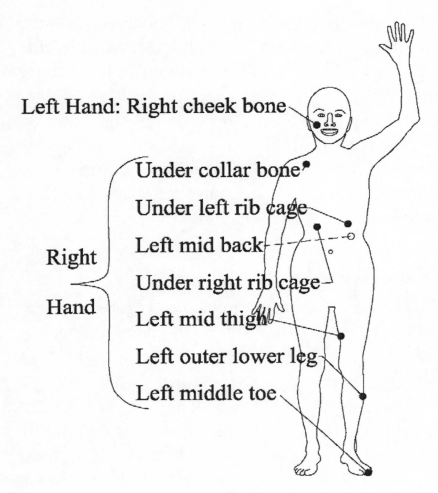

Left Hand: Right cheek bone

Under collar bone

Under left rib cage

Left mid back

Right

Under right rib cage

Hand

Left mid thigh

Left outer lower leg

Left middle toe

Figure 26

The sequence shown in Figure 26 is used starting with left hand on the right cheek bone and right hand under right collar bone. Left hand stays on cheek during the whole sequence. Right hand then moves to under left rib cage, then to left mid back, then to under right rib cage, then to left mid thigh, then to left outer lower leg, and finally to left middle toe.

This sequence can also be used starting with right hand on left cheek bone. Left hand goes under left collar bone, then to under right rib cage, then to right mid back, then to under left rib cage, then to right mid thigh, then to right outer lower leg, and finally to right middle toe.

For Jaw tension and tooth pain

Right jaw: Hold left hand over side of right jaw and hold right hand under right collar bone, see Figure 26.

Left jaw: Hold right hand over side of left jaw and hold left hand under left collar bone.

With one hand hold tense jaw and with other hand hold outside of opposite ankle.

Arms

Place left hand around right elbow or right upper arm to help elbow tension or pain (Burmeister, 1985a, 1981).

Place right hand around left upper arm or elbow for upper arm and elbow tension or pain. Placing the hands around the elbows helps us to realize our leadership and authority and helps relieve tension around the waistline.

For feeling tired

To help energize the body, use the sequence in Figure 27 below (Burmeister, 1985a, pp.41-42). Place left hand on inside of left ankle. Place right hand on tail bone. Then move left hand to under right rib cage. Then move right hand to left 3rd rib. Then move right hand to under right collar bone.

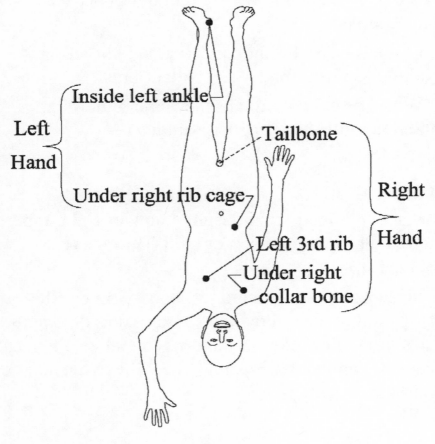

Figure 27

To use this same sequence on the other side of the body, start with the right hand on the right inside ankle and left hand on the tail bone. Then right hand moves to under left rib cage. Then left hand moves to right 3rd rib and then to under left collar bone.

This sequence helps enthusiasm, immune system, tongue, stomach, hiccups, proper functioning of body secretions and leg swelling.

For sciatic pain or tight hips

For right hip: Stand on left leg. Hold onto back of chair with left hand. Allow the right leg to be as loose as a puppet's leg with a string on the knee pulling the leg up. Swing right foot and leg in front in a large circle and then behind in large circle as shown in Figure 28 below:

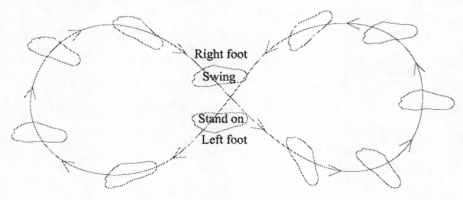

Figure 28

For left hip: Stand on right leg. Hold onto back of chair with right hand. Allow left leg to be loose. Swing left foot and leg in front in a large circle and then behind in a large circle as shown in Figure 29 below. Swing left leg freely in widest circles possible.

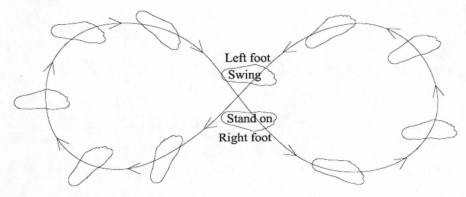

Figure 29

. Often pain in the hips, lower back and legs may result from too much sitting which tightens up all the muscles involved. This exercise shown in Figure 28 and Figure 29 loosens up the muscles connecting the sacrum to the leg, hip to leg, vertebrae to leg, and along the leg.

For tension in upper back and breasts

Right side: With left hand, hold upper right arm. With right hand, hold inner side of left knee (Burmeister, 1981). See Figure 30 below.

Left side: With right hand, hold upper left arm. With left hand, hold inner side of right knee.

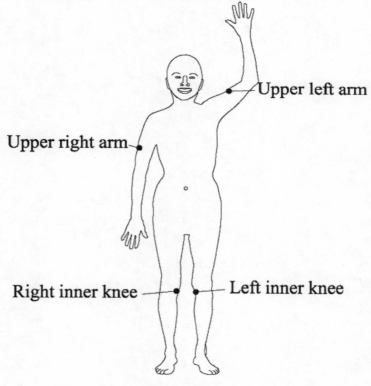

Figure 30

This combination of holding upper arm and opposite knee helps to relieve tension between shoulder blades, in the arms, knees, and also releases daily stress. To help with breast lumps, use this 3 times a day 20 minutes each time.

For skin: burns, sores, irritations

Place palm side of hands on back of lower legs just below knees (Burmeister, 1985a, p.54). See Figure 31 below.

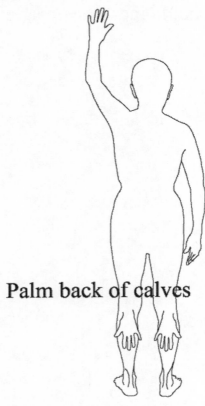

Palm back of calves

Figure 31

Palming the calves for 20 minutes 3 times a day can clear up many skin conditions. Palming the calves has helped healing of skin lesions. Continuous palming of the calves after burns can help skin to heal.

Lower back tension

While lying down and before eating, use hands to massage abdomen. Start at the outer edge of the abdomen under the rib cage, move fingers in a clockwise motion pressing gently into the abdomen. Massage the abdomen with small circles until the whole abdomen has been covered. By relaxing the abdominal muscles, the back is also relaxed.

The psoas muscle (lies along each side of the spine underneath the intestine, see Figure 32) may be in spasm; you can access this muscle by placing the fingertips deep into the side of the abdomen (in the area between rib cage and top of hip); the intestines will move out of the way. Then bend that knee up slowly while you have your fingertips in the abdomen; you will feel the psoas muscle contract when the knee comes up and lengthen when the knee goes down; bend the knee up and down slowly a few times. The psoas muscle relaxes and releases the sacroiliac joint. Relaxation of the psoas will also release lower back spasm in the lumbar region. Relax psoas muscle on the right as well as the one on the left. Breathe into the back.

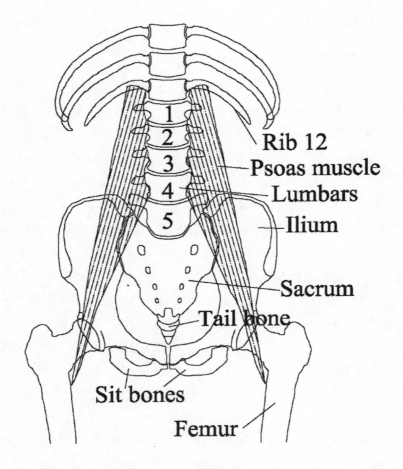

Figure 32

Figure 32 shows left and right psoas muscles, origin of each psoas muscle from 12th rib, lumbar vertebrae 1-4 to insertion on lesser trochanter of femur.

To help sinuses

Right sinuses: Place one hand on left side of back of neck. Place other hand on right forehead, then on right cheekbone close to nose, then under right collar bone close to midline of body. See Figure 33.

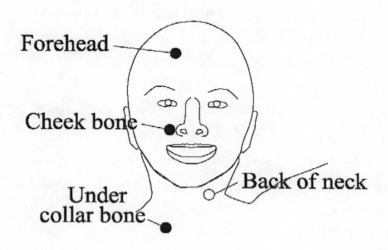

Figure 33

Left sinuses: Place one hand on right side of back of neck. Place other hand on left forehead, then on left cheekbone close to nose, then under left collar bone close to midline of body.

Fingers and Toes

For major projects such as diagnoses of different diseases, holding fingers and toes (Burmeister, 1985b) will help: 1) Right hand holds left thumb and at the same time left hand holds your right little toe for 3 minutes. 2) Then right hand holds left index finger and left hand holds right toe 4 (next to little toe) for 3 minutes. 3) Then right hand holds left middle finger and left hand holds right middle toe for 3 minutes. 4) Then right hand holds left ring finger (next to little finger) and left hand holds right toe 2 (next to big toe) for 3 minutes. 5) Then right hand holds left little finger and left hand holds right big toe. This finger-toe combination takes 15 minutes. You may also start by holding the little finger and big toe combination if you like.

Repeat holding right fingers and left toes: use your left hand to hold right fingers and use your right hand to hold left toes, for 3 minutes each. This combination also takes 15 minutes.

Repeat holding fingers and toes 3 times a day about 8 hours apart.

Figures 34 a, b, c, d, e, f show the energy pathways from left fingers to right toes. Figures 34 a, b, c show energy pathways from thoracic vertebrae 1-5, left back, back surface of left arm, hand and fingers to bottom of right foot and bottom of toes. Figures 34 d, e, f show energy pathways from sternum, front of left chest, front of left arm, left palm and fingers to front of right leg, top of right foot and top of toes.

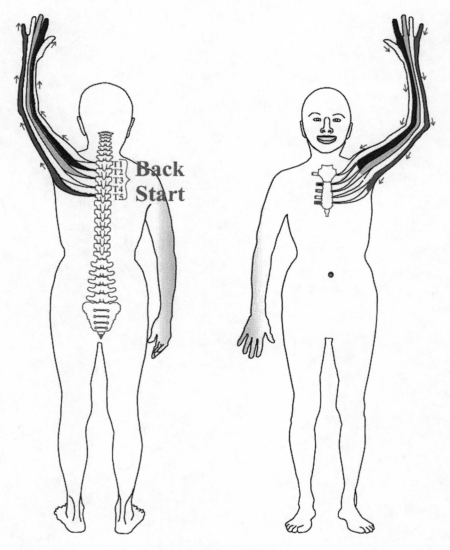

Figure 34a

Starting at thoracic vertebrae 1-5 the energy pathways go up left side of back, up back of left arm, up back of left hand over fingertips, down palm side of left hand, down front of left arm, deep into left chest, through sternum to right chest.

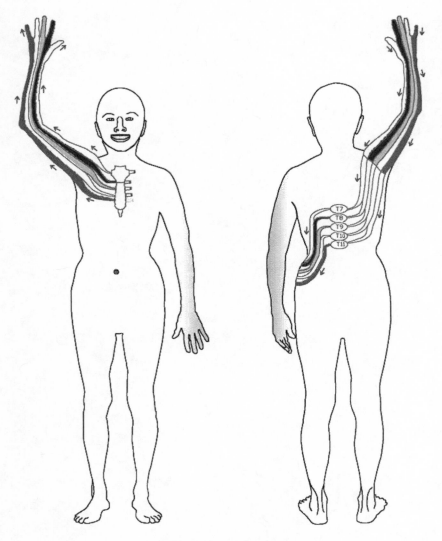

Figure 34 b

From surface of right chest goes across to front of right arm, to fingers, over fingertips, down back of right fingers, down back of right arm, goes deep diagonally through right back, through thoracic vertebrae 7-11, crossing diagonally down surface of left back.

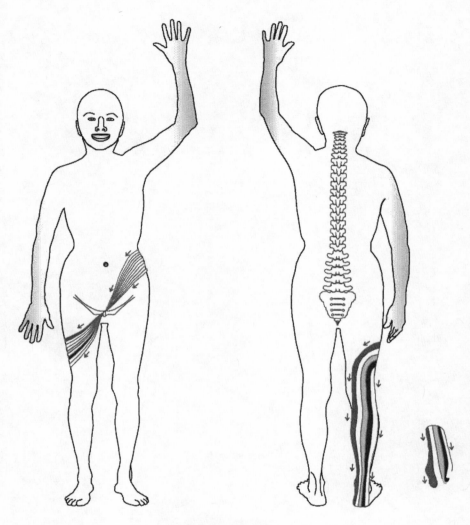

Figure 34 c

Goes diagonally deep into left abdomen toward pubic bone, spirals 180 degrees at pubic bone and continues diagonally across right front thigh surface toward lateral thigh. Wraps around lateral side of right leg and goes down back of right leg, through bottom surface of right foot.

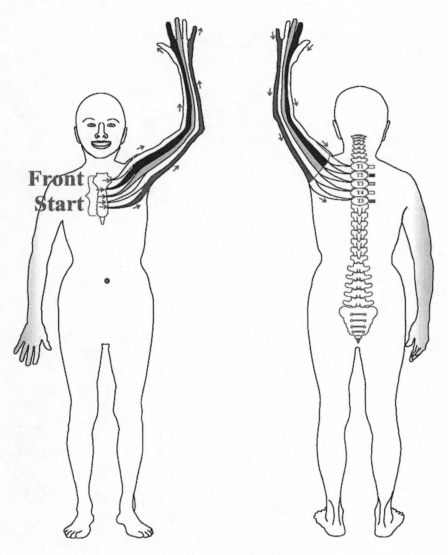

Figure 34 d

Begins at sternum, goes across surface of left chest, up front left arm, up palm and fingers, over fingertips. Down back side of left fingers, down back left arm, goes deep across left back, through thoracic vertebrae 1-5 area to right back surface.

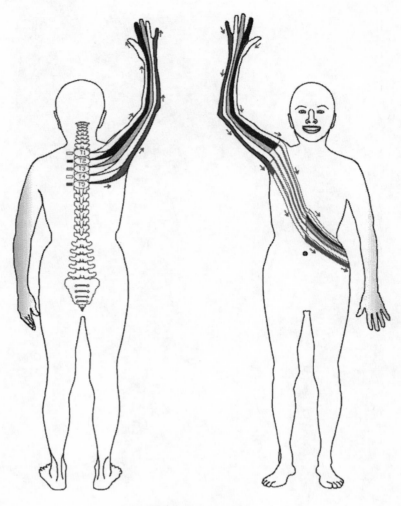

Figure 34e

From thoracic vertebrae 1-5 energy pathways go across right back surface, up back of right arm, up back of right hand and fingers, over fingertips. Down palm side of fingers and hand, down front of right arm, diagonally deep through right chest coming to the surface in left front abdomen, wrap on around to side of left hip.

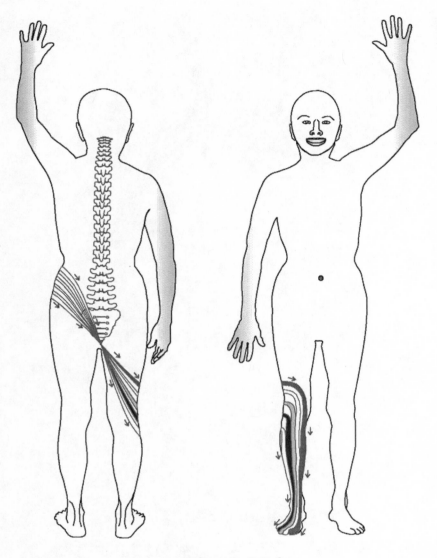

Figure 34 f

Energy pathways go deep in left hip toward tailbone, making a 180 degree turn there, then diagonally crossing back surface of right thigh; then wrapping around lateral thigh/knee to front of right lower leg continuing down top of foot ending in toes.

Holding the combination of fingers and toes helps all the structures along the paths of these invisible energies circulating through the body: ribs, arms, fingers, lungs, sternum, vertebrae, intestines, reproductive organs, legs, feet, heart, stomach, hip, muscles, skin surface, and joints. The energy pathways that start at left back (Figure 34 a) and left front (Figure 34 d) that go through: left thumb end in the right foot little toe, left index finger end in right toe 4, left middle finger end in right middle toe, left ring finger end in right toe 2, and left little finger end in right big toe.

An example of what is helped by holding left little finger and right big toe is heart function. From the back, the energy pathway starts at thoracic vertebra #5, goes to left little finger, goes through deep in the left chest, which includes the heart, and ends in the right big toe. If you cannot reach the right big toe, then just hold the left little finger. That goes for any of the finger – toe combinations.

There are similar pathways that start at right back and right front going through right fingers that end in left toes.

If symptoms or pain persist, consult your physician. The exercises described here are to help you in the healing process and maintain your health.

The Power to Heal

We can help ourselves any time, anywhere, just hold a finger. If that is not possible, then be present with the breath, let go of all worries and fears, smile and be thankful to be alive.

We are each basically good and want to behave in a loving way. However, we live in a society that values what we show on the outside: our appearance, the material world full of our possessions, our money, prestige and power. We start comparing and competing because we are fearful we do not have enough. When we are immersed in worry, fear, anger, sadness, or pretense, we become disconnected from our true selves and we go to places in the mind that detract from who we are. These disharmonies keep us from being present. Then instead of enjoying our life right now, we are suffering. We do not have to acquire more and more to be happy. We need to look within. Joy and happiness have always been present within us.

When we honor what is within us, we are connected to our soul and then the power to heal is available. When we are healed, we are not healed alone. All those around us also benefit from our healing. The harmony spreads. As more and more of us live from our soul as compassionate and kind human beings, we form a community of peaceful people.

References

Burmeister, Mary, 1985a, *Introducing Jin Shin Jyutsu Is, Book I*, Jin Shin Jyutsu, Inc., Scottsdale, AZ, 59pp.

Burmeister, Mary, 1981, *Introducing Jin Shin Jyutsu Is, Book II*, Jin Shin Jyutsu, Inc., Scottsdale, AZ, 68pp.

Burmeister, Mary, 1985b, *Introducing Jin Shin Jyutsu Is, Book III*, Jin Shin Jyutsu, Inc., Scottsdale, AZ, 42pp.

Heline, Corinne, 1940, *Occult Anatomy and the Bible*, New Age Press, Black Mountain, NC, 365pp.

Hirschi, Gertrud, 2000, *Mudras Yoga in your Hands*, Weiser, York Beach, ME, 230pp.

Ladinsky, Daniel, 1999, *The Gift Poems by Hafiz the Great Sufi Master*, Penguin Compass, New York, NY, 333pp.

Larsen, William J., 2001, *Human Embryology*, Third edition, Churchill Livingston, Philadelphia, PA, 548pp.

Netter, Frank H., 1989, *Atlas of Human Anatomy*, Second edition, Novartis, E. Hanover, NJ, 525plates.

Rolf, Ida P., 1977, *Rolfing Reestablishing the Natural Alignment and Structural Integration of the Human Body for Vitality and Well-Being*, Healing Arts Press, Rochester, VT, 304pp.

Smolan, Rick, Moffitt, Phillip, and Naythons, Matthew, 1990, *The Power to Heal Ancient Arts and Modern Medicine,* Prentice Hall Press, New York, NY, 224pp.

Yutang, Lin, 1937, *The Importance of Living*, Reynal and Hitchcock, New York, 459pp.

Index

jaw tension	79
jet lag	28,29
joints	70,71,87ff
kidney	41ff
knee	77ff,83
large intestine	55ff
legs	70,71,75,80,81,82,87ff
liver	48ff
lung	55ff,87ff
Main Central	69ff
memory	70,71
mouth	77ff
mudras	16ff
neck tension	76,77ff
nose	77ff
psoas muscle	85,86
pretense	63ff
reproductive system	70,71,87ff
ribs	87ff
sadness	22,23,54ff
sciatic pain	81,82
shoulder	73,74,75,83
sinuses	87

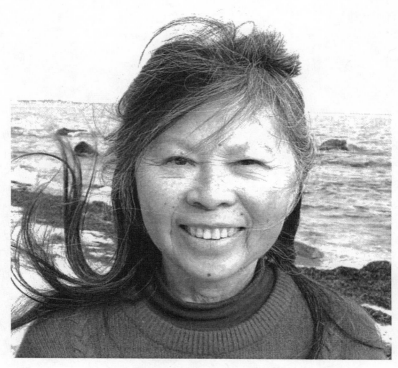

About the author

Betty Jean Wall was born to Chinese immigrant parents in a small town in Louisiana and grew up there asking many questions. She was trained as a biologist receiving her Ph.D. from University of Pittsburgh and worked for many years doing research in various institutions, including University of Cambridge, England, Case Western Reserve University, Cleveland, OH, University of Copenhagen, Denmark, Northwestern University, Evanston, IL, and Marine Biological Laboratory in Woods Hole, MA. Since 1980 she started studying the healing arts, including Jin Shin Jyutsu and Rolfing, learning how to help herself and others.